The Art of
HERBS FOR
HEALTH

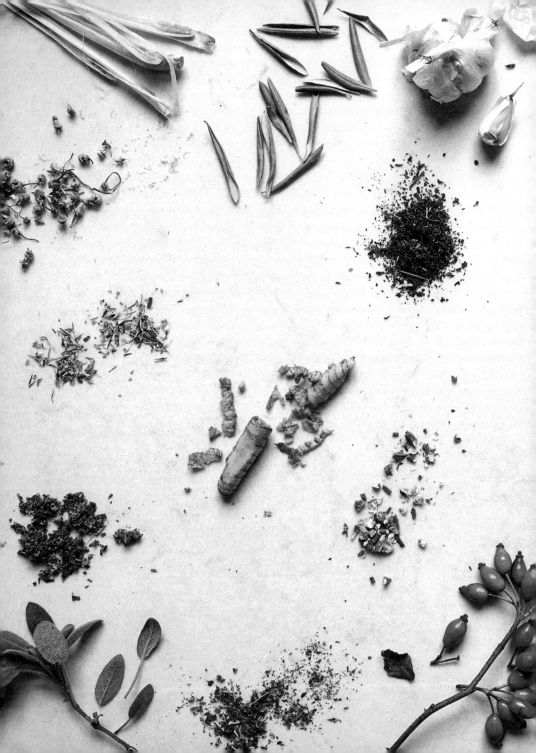

The Art of
HERBS FOR
HEALTH

Treatments, tonics and natural home remedies

Rebecca Sullivan

photography by Nassima Rothacker

Kyle Books

For the handiest herb handler I know, the greatest gardener of them all and a dear friend, Costa. Love your face.

An Hachette UK Company
www.hachette.co.uk

First published in Great Britain in 2018 by
Kyle Books, an imprint of Kyle Cathie Limited
Carmelite House, 50 Victoria Embankment
London EC4Y 0DZ
www.kylebooks.co.uk

10 9 8 7 6 5 4 3 2

ISBN 978 0 85783 477 5

Distributed in the US by Hachette Book Group,
1290 Avenue of the Americas, 4th and 5th Floors,
New York, NY 10104

Distributed in Canada by Canadian Manda
Group, 664 Annette St.,
Toronto, Ontario,
Canada, M6S 2C8

Project Editor: Tara O'Sullivan
Copy Editor: Anne Sheasby
Editorial Assistant: Sarah Kyle
Designer: Laura Woussen
Photographer: Nassima Rothacker
Illustrator: Chrissy Lau
Stylists: Rebecca Sullivan and Rachel de Thample
Prop Stylist: Agathe Gits
Production: Lisa Pinnell

A Cataloguing in Publication record for this title is
available from the British Library.

Printed and bound in China

The information and advice contained in this book are intended as a general guide to using plants and are not specific to individuals or their particular circumstances. Many plant substances, whether sold as foods or as medicines and used externally or internally, can cause an allergic reaction in some people. Neither the author nor the publishers can be held responsible for claims arising from the inappropriate use of any remedy or healing regime. Do not attempt self-diagnosis or self-treatment for serious or long-term conditions before consulting a medical professional or qualified practitioner. Do not undertake any self-treatment while taking other prescribed drugs or receiving therapy without first seeking professional guidance. Always seek medical advice if any symptoms persist.

CONTENTS

Introduction

One of my earliest memories is of watching my cat eat the green herbs and grasses in our backyard. I always thought she was a total weirdo, but she was actually doing something that all animals do. She was dispensing her own medicine, so to speak.

Herbs are incredible. They provide flavour, medicine and fragrance. Whilst the definition of a herb is any plant with leaves, seeds or flowers used for flavouring food, as medicine or as perfume, sometimes the line becomes a bit blurred. In this book, I have written recipes based on the three things that most people use, being flavour, medicine and scent, but I have also gone one step further and written these recipes with health in mind. However, please bear in mind that I am not a doctor, nor am I a person who is going to tell you that by using this book you will be a pillar of health and well-being and probably go onto Instagram success with a following of millions, have a body like a supermodel and a line of health products stocked in fancy stores.

What I am going to share with you though, are a few little things I have learned through working in the food industry for thirteen years, studying herbal medicine and turning my home into an apothecary in the meantime. I am going to share recipes I have learned from my elders – the ones who would never have just gone to get a prescription for antibiotics at the first sign of a cough. They didn't use paracetamol, ibuprofen or one of the numerous different brands of headache pills on offer. They didn't visit aisles in the supermarket dedicated solely to vitamins, omegas and food supplements. Instead they had gardens and allotments. They had herbs. They had, and of course still do have, plenty of common sense.

Those elders still use all these amazing skills and knowledge, the things I call granny skills, because they really work. And these skills and knowledge don't just work, they save us money and bring us closer to our land and the people around us. Let's use food as medicine. Don't ditch your doctor, don't avoid seeking advice, just look after yourself and your planet, and start to use the many wonderful things growing in your own backyard a little more often…

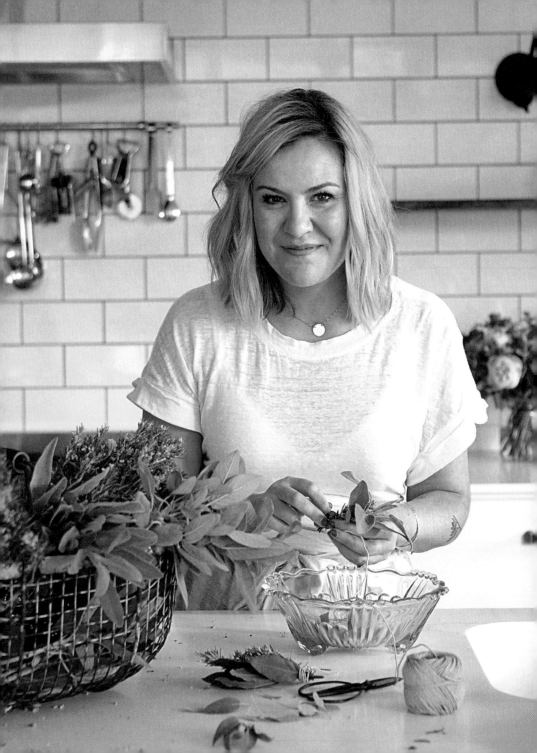

Herb guide

Below is a list of common medicinals that are food/culinary herbs and what parts to eat.

Anise Hyssop (*Agastache foeniculum*) – flowers, stems and leaves

Basil (*Ocimum spp.*) – flowers, stems and leaves

Bay (*Laurus nobilis*) – leaves

Bee Balm (*Monarda*) – flowers, stems and leaves

Borage (*Borago officinalis*) – flower and young leaves

Calendula (*Calendula officinalis, Asteraceae*) – petals and young leaves

Chervil (*Anthriscus cerefolium*) – stems and leaves

Chickweed (*Stellaria media, Caryophyllaceae*)

Chives (*Allium Schoenoprasum*) – bulbs, flowers and leaves

Dandelion (*Taraxacum officinale, Asteraceae*) – roots, flowers and leaves

Dill (*Anethum graveolens*) – flowers, stems and leaves

Elderberry (*Sambucus nigra, Adoxaceae*) – flowers and berries

Fennel (*Foeniculum vulgare*)

Hawthorn (*Crataegus spp., Rosaceae*)

Hibiscus (*Hibiscus sabdariffa, Malvaceae*)

Lemon Balm (*Melissa officinalis*) – flowers, stems and leaves

Marjoram (*Origanum majorana*) – flowers, stems and leaves

Mint (*Mentha spp.*) – flowers, stems and leaves

Oregano (*Origanum vulgare*) – flowers, stems and leaves

Parsley (*Petroselinum crispum*) – roots, flowers, stems and leaves

Peppermint (*Mentha piperita*) – flowers, stems and leaves

Rosemary (*Rosmarinus officinallis*) – flowers, stems and leaves

Sage (*Salvia spp.*) – flowers, stems and leaves

Tarragon (*Artemisia dracunculus*) – flowers, stems and leaves

Thyme (*Thymus spp.*) – flowers, stems and leaves

Tulsi (*Ocimum tenuiflorum, Lamiaceae*)

Violet (*Viola sororia, Violaceae*) – flowers, stems and leaves

White sage (*Salvia apiana*) – flowers, stems and leaves

Wild garlic (*Allium ursinum*) – roots, flowers, stems and leaves

When & where to grow herbs

Herbs grow best with full sun and light, in well-drained, moisture-retentive, fertile soil with plenty of organic nutrients and compost incorporated.

- Choose several cultivars, where available, with different harvesting times to help keep the herb garden productive and available all year round.
- Pot up herbs grown outdoors, such as chives, mint, parsley or tarragon, and bring them in for the winter, standing them on a south-facing windowsill.
- Plant up larger containers with stronger-growing herbs, such as mint and sage, and pot up smaller ones for your kitchen or windowsill for easy picking.
- Start sowing herbs early in the spring.
- Sow a few trays in a greenhouse, conservatory or sunny windowsill and grow plants on ready for planting out once the soil is warmer.
- Herb and salad gardens make a great gift and don't need to be huge. Choose a few herbs that complement each other and plant in an old container or large bowl with some holes for drainage.

Warnings

Foraging for herbs and flowers for medicines and food can be one of the most exciting and rewarding experiences, but there are a few rules that really should be adhered to out of respect to our environment, biodiversity and our neighbours (the birds and bees).

- Pick only what you need and always, always leave some behind.
- Be absolutely positive of your identification before you harvest and ingest any wild food or medicine. It is common sense that you should know what you are harvesting. If in doubt, do not pick!
- Consult with local herbalists, botanists and experts. Be especially careful with plants in families that contain deadly poisonous members, such as the carrot (*Apiaceae*) and buttercup (*Ranunculaceae*) families. Positively identify it at least three times before you pick it.

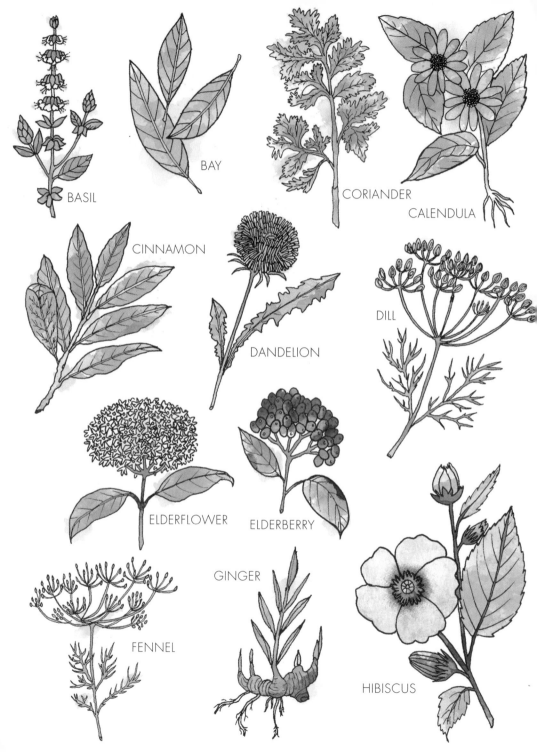

BASIL

BAY

CORIANDER

CALENDULA

CINNAMON

DANDELION

DILL

ELDERFLOWER

ELDERBERRY

GINGER

FENNEL

HIBISCUS

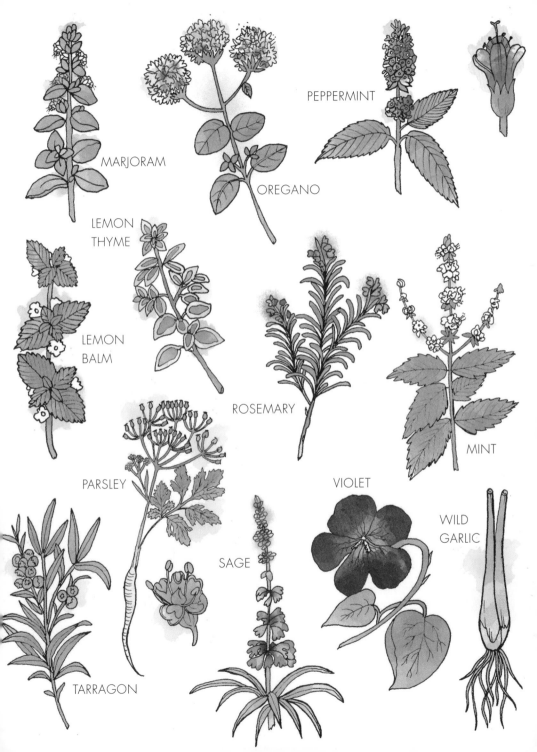

MARJORAM

OREGANO

PEPPERMINT

LEMON
THYME

LEMON
BALM

ROSEMARY

MINT

PARSLEY

VIOLET

WILD
GARLIC

TARRAGON

SAGE

A bit about herbal teas

My partner Damien and I have an Indigenous Australian brand called *Warndu*, which in his language means 'Good'. Our hero products are our herbal teas using Native Australian ingredients. The process of developing these teas was absolutely incredible and I learnt so much about the power of herbs, in particular our Native herbs, which are superfoods. To add to this I decided to study herbal medicine (a short course) so I could learn more about how they all work together in harmony.

Needless to say I am now a herbal tea lover. I sip on it all day, everyday. Its many combinations have all kinds of abilities, from aiding in digestion, helping you sleep to calming your nerves. Below is a little list of my favourite herbs and spices to help with common everyday ailments and symptoms. Use the below dried in a teapot or using a strainer with some boiling water. I would work to half a teaspoon per ingredient per cup of water bearing in mind some of them are much stronger than others so just experiment. And remember to test them in small quantities first for allergies.

ANGELICA

Great for digestion, irritable bowel syndrome (IBS), gas and anything to do with your digestion. It also acts as an anti-inflammatory, so it can help with arthritis.

BURDOCK

A blood cleanser, diuretic and used to treat eczema, arthritis and gout.

CALENDULA

Can be used internally and externally – wonderful for rashes, wounds and burns. Helps with ulcers, reflux and is antimicrobial.

CHAMOMILE

Well known for its ability to assist in sleep and can also help with anxiety and stress.

CHICKWEED

Acts as a blood cleanser and is good for iron deficiency.

DANDELION

A perfect all rounder and widely available. The root encourages healthy gut and can stimulate digestion. Dandelion can also have a liver cleansing effect.

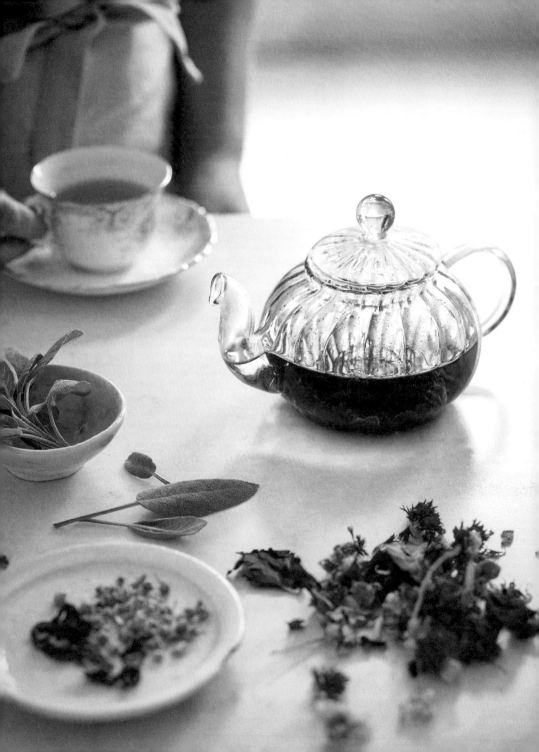

ECHINACEA

Wards off colds and flu. It stimulates our immune system so our bodies can fight infections quicker.

GARLIC

A potent tonic for boosting circulation and fighting off colds and flu. Best to avoid if you suffer from heartburn or are prone to gas.

GINGER

An amazing all rounder for motion sickness, nausea, digestion, infection and to boost circulation.

HIBISCUS OR ROSELLE

Has antimicrobial properties and helps with high cholesterol and lowering blood pressure. Also great for the liver and kidneys.

HOLY BASIL OR TULSI

A remedy for colds and flu, sinus infections and can also help with anxiety, asthma and coughs. It is also said to be beneficial for improving concentration and poor memory.

LEMON BALM

Helpful for depression and anxiety and also wonderful for unwinding and aiding in inducing sleep. Mild enough for children and elders.

LEMONGRASS

Helpful for headaches, stress, coughs, indigestion and menstrual cramps.

LEMON VERBENA

Good for nausea and insomnia. Mild enough for children and elders.

LIQUORICE

Good for heartburn, irritable bowel syndrome (IBS), sore throat, coughs and tendonitis.

NETTLES

Packed with vitamins, minerals and chlorophyll, nettles help with tiredness and tension.

MARSHMALLOW

Recommended for whooping cough and bronchitis.

PEPPERMINT/MINT

Good for digestion.

RASPBERRY LEAF

Good for cold sores, anaemia and morning sickness.

ROSE

Pink and red rose petals are high in bioflavonoids, which are antioxidant and anti-inflammatory.

ROSEMARY

This has antibacterial and antioxidant properties.

TURMERIC

A magical anti-inflammatory and antioxidant. Great for arthritis, pain and achy muscles. On its own, turmeric is poorly absorbed in the bloodstream, and needs to be blended with black pepper to be effective.

VALERIAN

Well known for insomnia and perfect too for menstrual cramps, headaches, aches and anxiety.

VIOLET

Can be used as a blood cleanser and is good for chest infections and dry coughs. There are hundreds of species of violets worldwide so check the Latin name (see page 10) to make sure it's edible before consuming.

WHITE SAGE

Good for easing congestion and respiratory issues. Also good for colds and flu.

YARROW

Anti-microbial and anti-inflammatory yarrow also helps with bruising, thread or spider veins and haemorrhoids.

Quick cures & herbal helpers

For when you don't have time to make a whole recipe, here are some simple herbal remedies to keep you feeling well.

Nausea

Add a 5cm piece of bruised fresh ginger to 500ml boiling water. Let it infuse overnight. Strain into ice cube trays and freeze until solid. Suck on them or add to your water glass when feeling nauseous.

Ear Ache

Peel a garlic clove and place into the sore ear canal (being careful not to push it in too far). Leave in overnight whilst you sleep. Do the same for colds by placing a peeled garlic clove in your sock (that you are wearing), tucking it in somewhere comfortable.

Smelly Feet

Make some really strong black tea in a bucket. Leave it to cool to touch and then soak your feet in it for about 30 minutes (whilst watching Netflix or reading a book). The tannins in tea get rid of bacteria.

Bad Breath

Gargle with a small cup of acidic lemon juice to kill odour-causing bacteria. Then eat a little unsweetened natural yogurt, which contains beneficial lactobacillus bacteria. These so-called probiotics compete with and replace the reeking bacteria.

Flatulence

Sip on peppermint tea. Peppermint kills the bacteria that causes bloating and relaxes your gastrointestinal muscles.

A bit about essential oils

Essential oils are the natural oils from all kinds of common things like lavender and orange peel (or in fancy terms a concentrated hydrophobic liquid containing volatile aroma compounds from plants). They are harvested and distilled (mostly using steam) down into a pure form or the aromatic compound. This is the pure essence of the stem of a plant, the root, bark, seed or flowers. Sure, they smell good, but what's behind the smell are some seriously magical organic compounds that, when used correctly, can become your first port of call for skin care, aromatherapy, ailments and illnesses, mental health and well-being.

There are three ways to use them

- diffused (aromatically)
- topically (on your skin)
- internally (tinctures, tonics and edibles)

I use a lot of essential oils in my books. I am by no means an expert, but I know that where I have used them, I have used them for a reason and because they have worked for me. They are an expensive addition to your staples but they last a long time so are an investment. But if they aren't in your budget don't fret, you can always sub it out or just use one instead of a blend for example. Like all things, try them on a small patch first to see if your skin can handle them or if you're allergic. Always check if they are for aromatic, topical or internal use before experimenting.

Chapter One
treatments

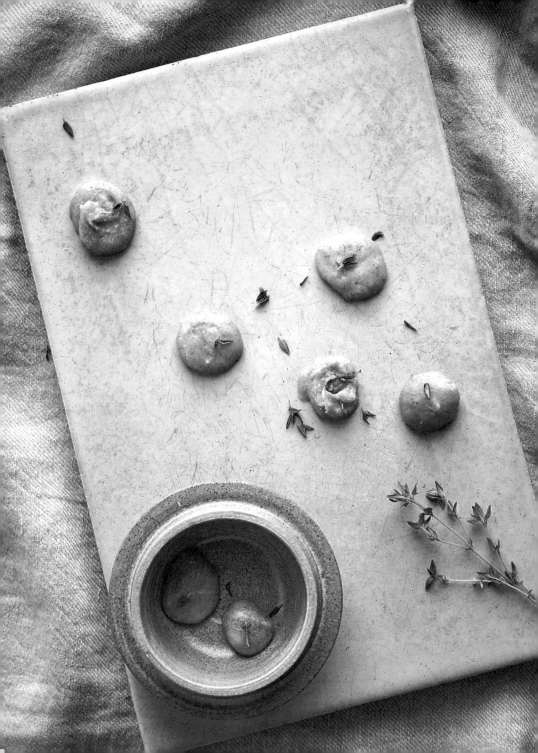

Once removed from the fridge, these will melt and lose their shape quickly – so keep them cool.

Honey & thyme throat lozenges

These little beauties taste unbelievably delicious – so much better than those fake, chemical-tasting cough drops you buy at the pharmacy. Admittedly these lozenges are a little sticky and gooey, but just keep them in the fridge and use as needed.

MAKES ABOUT 20

60ml coconut oil

60ml raw honey

½ teaspoon ground cinnamon

1cm piece of fresh ginger, peeled and grated

sprig of lemon thyme, leaves picked and chopped

small ice cube trays

Place the coconut oil in a bowl and beat with a hand-held mixer (or use a stand mixer) until it's whipped. Add the honey and continue to whip until they are combined. Add the cinnamon, ginger and lemon thyme and mix again. Pour the mixture into the smallest ice cube trays you can find or half-fill larger ones – you want to create bite-sized lozenges.

Freeze for about 40 minutes until they're hard. Pop them out of the ice cube trays and store in an airtight container in the fridge until needed. These lozenges will keep in the fridge for up to 10 days.

Herbal honey cough medicine

Honey provides so many benefits, from antibacterial to anti-inflammatory. When the season turns cold, the dreaded coughs and colds begin. A sore throat can mean sleepless nights, and one of the simplest solutions is honey. It acts in a similar way to cough syrup by coating the throat and soothing it. Add herbs to that and you have your very own natural cough syrup. Use it in your teas as a herbal sweetener or take a tablespoon before bed or when necessary.

Make as much as you like at a time. Try any of the following dried herbs, spices and fruits:

angelica root

calendula

echinacea

elderberry

hawthorn berries

lemon balm and lemon verbena
  (a mix of the two)

rose petals

turmeric root and black
  peppercorns (just a few)

garlic (4–5 cloves)

raw honey

sterilised jar large enough to fit the
  amount you make

You can either use shop-bought dried or home grown and dried herbs. Just ensure they are ground reasonably finely using your mortar and pestle or in a food-processor. Mix equal proportions of honey with the herbs (so 100g honey to 100g dried herbs).

Place the honey and herb mix in a double boiler and keep over a low heat for 6 hours, ensuring that the honey doesn't exceed 43–46°C. If you don't have a double boiler, then you can easily make one at home by placing a smaller pan inside a larger one, using jar lid rings or a trivet to keep the inner pan off the bottom of the larger pan. Stir the mix every now and then so it infuses evenly, remembering that you may need to add more water to the pan due to evaporation.

After 6 hours, strain the honey while it is still warm, using a muslin cloth, or a piece of tighter weave muslin, or even a clean cotton T-shirt is fine. Press the mix through the material, wringing it until it has all come through. Pour into a sterilised jar and seal. Label and store in a cool, dark place for up to a year. Once opened, keep at room temperature.

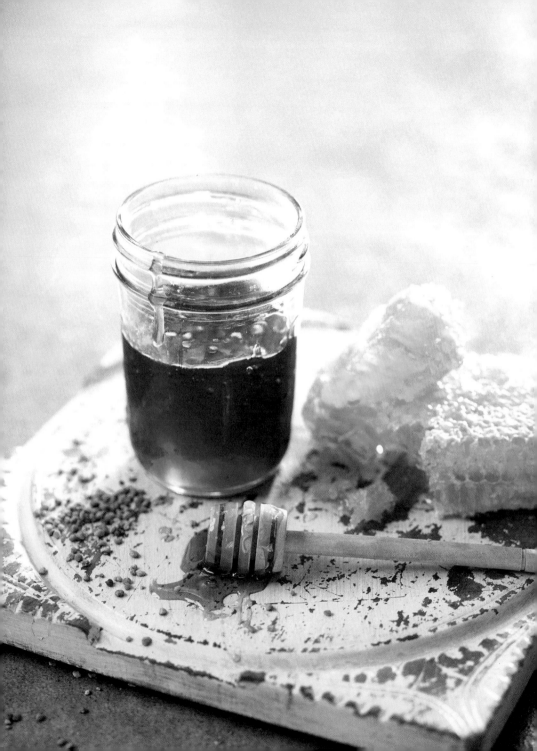

Sore throat spray

Don't wait for it to develop into an actual sore throat. At the first sign of a tickle, spray your throat with this spray, and even if it's not a sore throat this is so perfectly natural that it doesn't matter.

MAKES 100ML

1 teaspoon dried echinacea
100ml boiling water
6 teaspoons raw honey

Sterilised 100ml spray bottle

Put the echinacea into a small heatproof bowl and pour over the boiling water. Leave it to steep for 5 minutes. Strain into a small jug, and then once it's coolish (not cold), stir in the honey. Pour into a small, sterilised spray bottle. Use at the first sign of a sore throat by spraying in your mouth. Use as needed. Store in the bathroom for a few months.

Some really excellent edible weeds

We are used to thinking of weeds as a bad thing, and people spend hours trying to rid their gardens of them. But they can, in fact, have fantastic medicinal uses. Here are a few to look out for:

Amaranth (*Amaranthus retroflexus*)
Burdock (*Arctium lappa*)
Chickweed (*Stellaria media*)
Dandelion (*Taraxacum officinalis*)
Garlic Mustard (*Alliaria officinalis*)
Lamb's Quarter (*Chenopodium album*)

Mallows (*Malva neglecta* and related species)
Purslane (*Portulacca oleracea*)
Queen Anne's Lace (*Daucus carota*)
Sheep Sorrel (*Rumex acetosella*)
Stinging Nettle (*Urtica dioica*)
Yellow Dock (*Rumex crispus*)

Ginger & peppermint travel sickness pastilles

Damien, my boyfriend, gets travel sickness a lot, the poor thing. I hated the thought of him eating the packets of travel sickness pills with all kinds of unpronounceable things in them, so these are jam-packed with the things that ease nausea – ginger and peppermint.

MAKES 20

500g fresh blackberries or raspberries, washed
2 medium cooking apples, peeled, diced and cored
juice of ½ lemon
5cm piece of fresh ginger, peeled and grated, or 2 teaspoons ground ginger
1 tablespoon dried peppermint
300g caster sugar

Line a deep 10–15cm square cake tin with baking paper and set aside.

Place the berries and apples into a saucepan and add the lemon juice and 150ml water. Bring to the boil, then reduce the heat and stir in the ginger and peppermint. Cover and simmer, stirring occasionally, for about 20–30 minutes until the fruit is tender.

Pass the mixture through a fine sieve into a large bowl, and use the back of a wooden spoon to push it through the sieve.

Return the purée to the pan, add the sugar, then heat gently, stirring frequently, until the sugar has dissolved. Bring to the boil, then reduce the heat and cook, stirring occasionally, for around 15–20 minutes until the mixture is very thick. As it thickens, stir more frequently so it doesn't burn.

Pour into the prepared tin, then leave to cool completely before removing and cutting into bite-sized pieces. Store in an airtight container in the fridge for up to a month.

Kombucha, liquorice, raspberry & mint gut jellies

A few of my favourite things all mixed together in wobbly little jelly slices. Kombucha is so incredible for gut health and the liquorice and mint help with digestion too, so these are an all round hug for your belly. Best eaten after a meal.

MAKES 20

500g fresh raspberries

1 litre kombucha

1 tablespoon raw honey

½ teaspoon ground liquorice root

2 tablespoons gelatine (I would strongly recommend checking the packet of the gelatine brand you use and follow instructions per litre of liquid here).

120ml filtered water, at room temperature

4 sprigs of mint, cut or ripped into small pieces

Line a 30cm rectangular or 23cm square shallow cake tin with clingfilm so it hangs over the edges for easy removal once set. Put the raspberries, kombucha, honey and liquorice root in a blender and blend until smooth. Pass the mixture through a fine sieve to remove any seeds – you can skip this step if you don't mind the seeds (which I don't). Place the mixture in a saucepan over a low heat and bring to a simmer, but do not boil.

Meanwhile, place the gelatine in a small bowl with the filtered water and whisk together, then leave to sit for 5 minutes. Add the soaked gelatine and water to the warm berry mixture and stir over a low heat until the gelatine is completely dissolved. Skim off any foam that is sitting on the top, if you like. Pour the mixture into the prepared tin, then leave to set in the fridge for at least 8 hours or overnight.

Once set, remove the slab of jelly (using the clingfilm to help), turn it out onto a chopping board and then cut into small cubes or use a small cutter to cut out bite-sized shapes. Store in an airtight container in the fridge until needed. These jellies will keep in the fridge for up to a week.

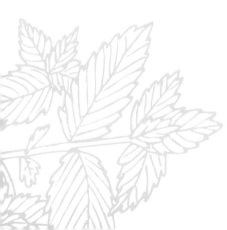

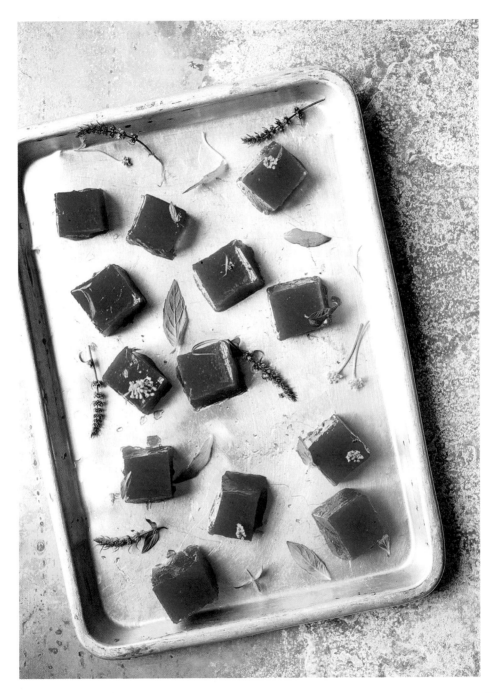

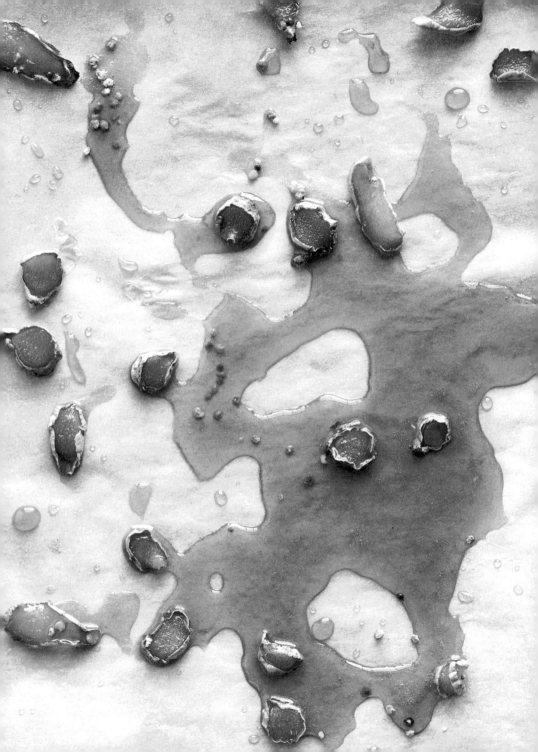

Ginger & basil digestion sweets

Not only good for digestion, this is another fabulous little candy for nausea and travel sickness, or indeed when you are feeling a little run down, as ginger is fabulous at fighting bugs and flus.

MAKES ABOUT 20

100g fresh ginger, sliced (I prefer it unpeeled, but you can peel it if you like)
100g raw honey
small bunch of fresh basil, chopped or a few drops of basil essential oil

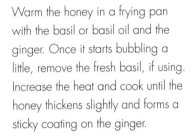

Warm the honey in a frying pan with the basil or basil oil and the ginger. Once it starts bubbling a little, remove the fresh basil, if using. Increase the heat and cook until the honey thickens slightly and forms a sticky coating on the ginger.

Spoon onto greaseproof paper to cool and dry a little. They'll still be sticky once dried but the honey should set further, making them easy to handle. Store in a box in the fridge for up to a month.

Decongestant rub (for colds & flu)

I'm not going to lie, I actually love the smell of Vicks vapour rub, but in the aim of having a DIY home, I had to give this a go myself and it really does work. The other beauty here is that when you put Vicks under your nose, it kind of burns; this does not! It's also great for headaches – just put a little on your temples and where the pain is on your forehead.

MAKES 150G

150g coconut oil

4 sprigs each of oregano, sage, thyme and basil, ripped into pieces

15 drops of thyme essential oil

15 drops of eucalyptus essential oil

15 drops of lavender essential oil

10 drops of lemon essential oil

Gently heat the coconut oil and all of the herbs in a double boiler until the oil begins to go slightly green. If you don't have a double boiler, simply place the coconut oil and herbs in a heatproof bowl over a saucepan of barely simmering water (ensuring the bottom of the bowl doesn't touch the water underneath).

Remove from the heat and leave to cool, then strain into a clean bowl or jug and stir in the essential oils. Transfer to a small, sterilised jar, seal and label. Store in the bathroom for up to 6 months. Use liberally when needed.

The temperature of your bathroom or medicine cabinet will affect whether the rub is liquid or solid. Either way, it is still fine to use.

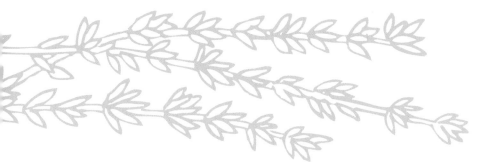

Herby chest rub (for asthma)

This one is for my little godson, Charlie. The poor little monkey is in and out of hospital so often with his asthma. I am hoping that once he gets over the scary young age for his asthma, he can use this as a preventer. It is also great if you have a cold too, and makes for a fab steam.

MAKES ABOUT 20G

15g beeswax
10 drops of thyme essential oil
10 drops of eucalyptus essential oil
10 drops of lavender essential oil
10 drops of frankincense
    essential oil

small sterilised jar

Gently heat the beeswax until melted, either in a double boiler or in a heatproof bowl over a saucepan of barely simmering water (ensuring the bottom of the bowl doesn't touch the water underneath).

Remove from the heat and leave to cool, then stir in the essential oils. Transfer to a small, sterilised jar, seal and label. Store in the bathroom for up to a a year. Use liberally when needed by rubbing into your chest.

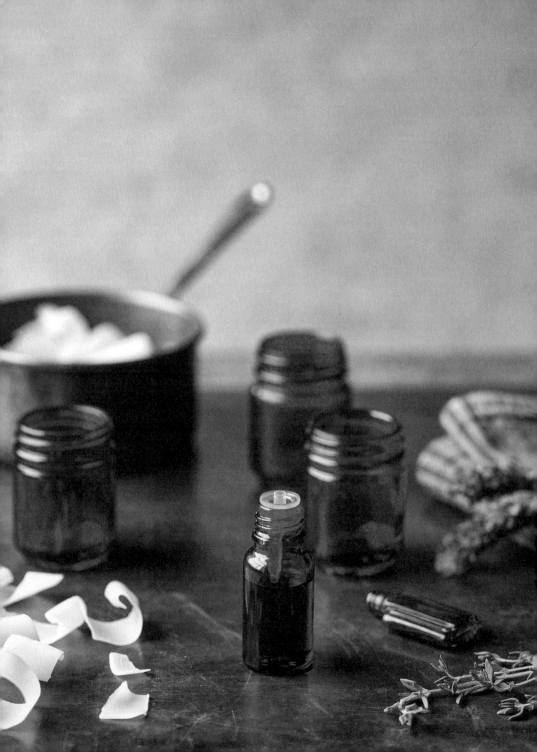

Flower & leaf stress balls

These make me so happy! Squeeze and smell. They really work. The blend of essential oils is chosen to reduce anxiety and induce calm using common things you have in your garden and bathroom. If you don't have essential oils, just use the fresh stuff and refresh it with new ones weekly (or more often if you have squished the life out of it after a particularly stressful day).

MAKES 1

5 drops of thyme essential oil
5 drops of eucalyptus essential oil
5 drops of lavender essential oil
5 drops of rosemary essential oil
4 cotton wool balls or pads
4 sprigs each of oregano, sage, thyme and basil, ripped into pieces
4 sprigs of lavender, ripped into pieces
a handful of dried rose petals

small square of muslin, cheesecloth or the end of an old stocking
piece of string

Put each type of essential oil onto an individual cotton wool ball or pad. Stuff them and all the herbs and flowers into the muslin, cheesecloth or stocking. Tie up securely with string and every time you are feeling a little stressed, squeeze and smell. Make a new one regularly to keep it fresh.

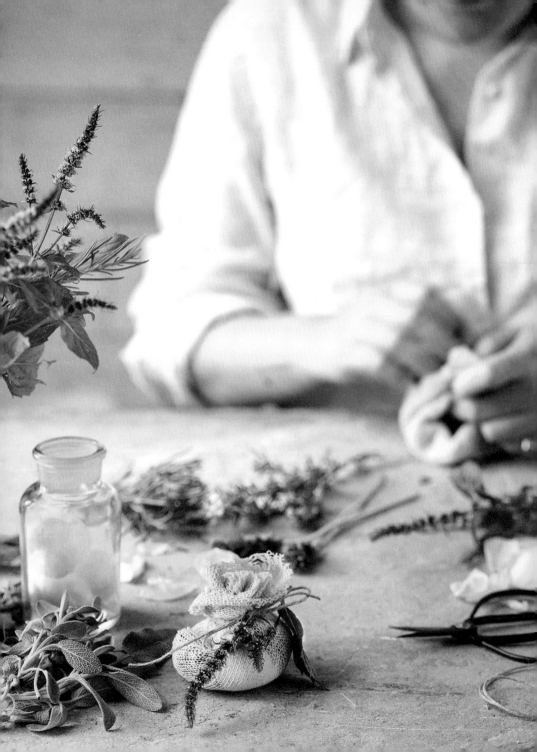

Chapter Two
drinks
& tonics

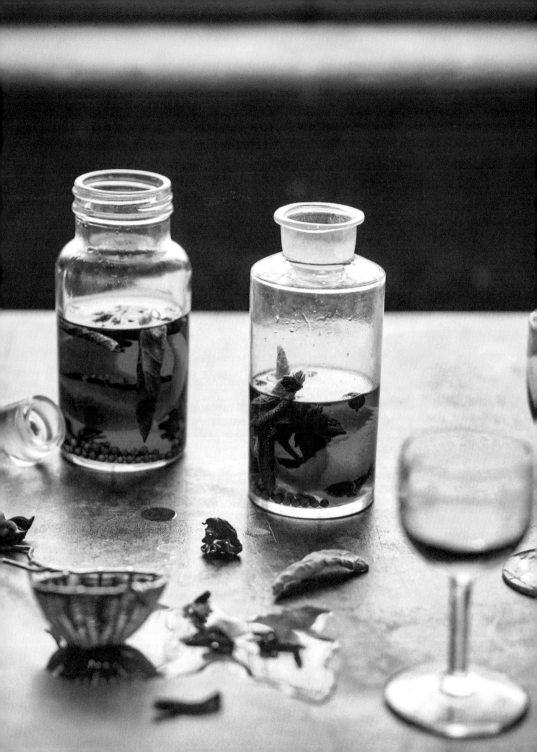

Herbal bitters

Bitters are said to curb sugar cravings, which in theory makes little sense to me – to curb *my* sugar cravings, I eat chocolate – but surprisingly, they actually work. They also make a fantastic addition to a cocktail, and if you happen to drink too many cocktails, they're fabulous for nausea – just take as a small shot or put it in your water bottle.

MAKES 250ML

1 pink grapefruit
1 blood orange
40g dried juniper berries
15g dried whole hibiscus flowers
4 tablespoons dried thyme
8 star anise
2 tablespoons dried mint
2 teaspoons ground white pepper
2 bay leaves
2 tablespoons honey
250ml brandy

sterilised 250ml jar

Cut the grapefruit and orange into squares and add to a sterilised jar, along with all the other ingredients. Seal and shake well. Label and store in a cool, dark place for six weeks to infuse – you can use it sooner, if you wish, but six weeks will allow the herbs to macerate and infuse. This will keep for up to two years.

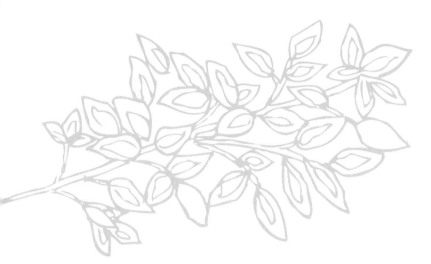

Herbal waters

Useful for cooking, beauty products, tinctures and tonics. These are also just lovely to spritz about the place for a quick whiff of herby delights. You can actually try this recipe with just about any herb you have growing at home, and the more herbs you use in the recipe, the stronger the water.

MAKES 200ML

200ml filtered water

6 tablespoons fresh or dried edible herbs of your choice, such as rosemary, sage, bay or lemon thyme

sterilised 200ml jar

Bring the water to the boil in a small saucepan. Place the herbs in a heatproof bowl. Pour over the boiling water and cover with a plate to weight it down. Leave to infuse overnight at room temperature.

Strain the water into a sterilised jar, then seal and store in the fridge for up to 6 months. Use as needed.

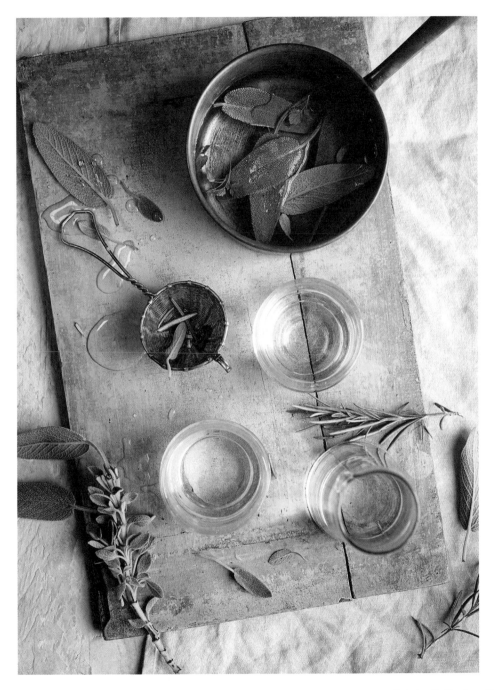

Try a combination of orange and rosemary, rose and mint or tarragon and raspberry.

Sage & lavender kefir

Kefir, much like kombucha and other fermented foods, is incredible at aiding good gut health. Unflavoured, it can be a little uninspiring, benefits aside. I love this combination of sage and lavender, but you can use this recipe as a base and make it your own with herbs that suit your tastes and needs.

MAKES 1 LITRE

4 tablespoons caster sugar

1 litre coconut water

2 tablespoons water kefir grains

sprig of sage

sprig of lavender

sprig of mint

slice of lemon

sterilised 1 litre jar or bottle

Mix the sugar into the coconut water until dissolved. Pour into a clean bowl, then add the kefir grains, sage, lavender, mint and lemon. Cover with a tea towel and leave to ferment in a cool, dark place for 2–3 days.

Strain through a clean cloth or muslin (don't use a metal sieve) into a sterilised jar, seal and store in the fridge. Drink within 3 weeks. It will taste tangy.

Thyme & orange blossom hot cacao

Try this warm in winter and over ice in summer for a brunch addition or afternoon pick-me-up. The thyme can be subbed out for rosemary or sage, if you prefer. Or, if you are feeling adventurous, use all three (just a third of each).

SERVES 2

250ml whole milk

250ml double cream

150g dark chocolate (70 per cent cocoa solids is best), broken into small pieces

1 sprig of thyme, leaves picked

2 teaspoons orange blossom water

1 tablespoon honey (optional)

1 tablespoon dried rose petals, to decorate

Put all the ingredients, except the rose petals, into a small pan and heat slowly until the chocolate melts completely, but don't let the mixture boil. Strain out the thyme leaves, pour into mugs and serve with rose petals sprinkled over as decoration.

For a dairy-free version, just switch out the cream and milk for your choice of nut, rice or oat milk.

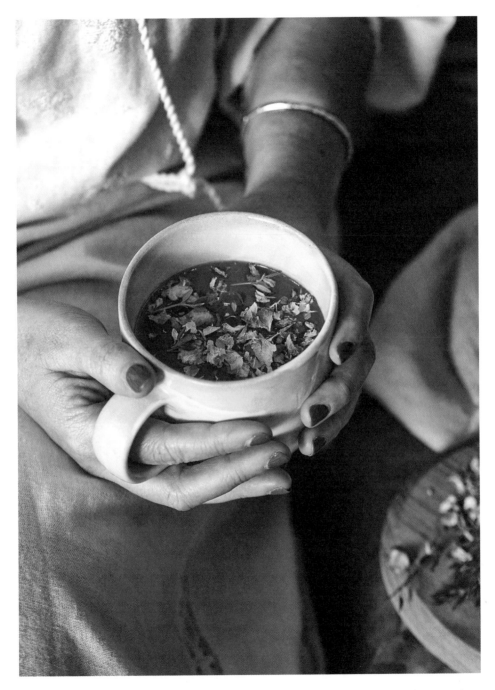

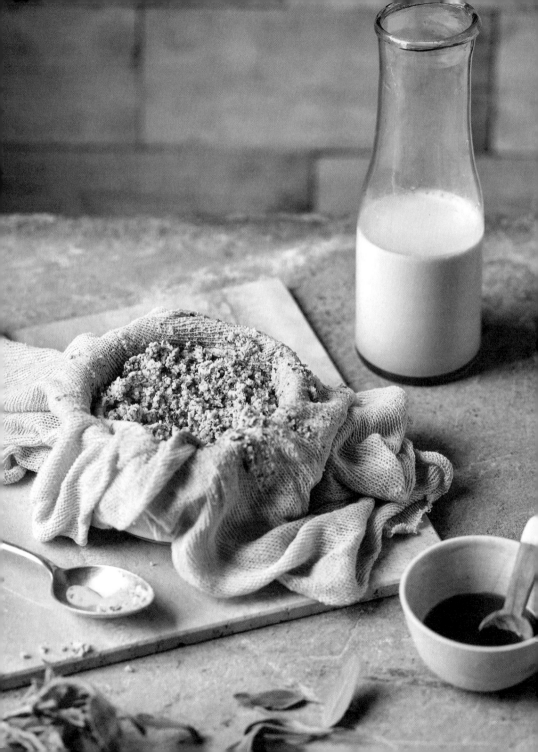

Almond, sage & honey milk

This is the most perfect dairy-free alternative to cow's milk. When it's then used in things like porridge or desserts you don't even need to add any other aromats and flavours as it's already flavourful.

MAKES 750ML–1 LITRE

500g raw (unblanched) whole almonds

1 litre filtered water, plus extra for pre-soaking

2 sprigs of sage, leaves picked

2–3 tablespoons raw honey, to taste

pinch of salt, or to taste

1 litre sterilised jar or glass bottle

Soak the almonds by placing them in a bowl and covering with about 5cm of extra filtered water. The almonds will absorb the water and expand. Cover the bowl with a tea towel and leave in a cool place overnight or in the fridge for a couple of days.

When you are ready to prepare your milk, drain and rinse the almonds. Slip off the skins of the almonds and discard (if you can be bothered!). Combine the almonds, 1 litre of filtered water and the sage in a high-speed blender. Pulse a few times to loosen the almonds, then blend at the highest speed for 2 minutes. Or, if you are using a food-processor, process for 4 minutes in total, pausing to scrape down the sides halfway through. The milk will look like a mix of fine meal and white opaque water.

Line a sieve with a piece of muslin or cheesecloth and place over a measuring jug. Pour the almond mixture into the sieve. Press all the almond milk from the almond meal – do this by gathering the cloth around the almond meal and twisting. Squeeze and press to extract as much almond milk as possible. Keep the almond meal for baking. You should get about 750ml–1 litre of milk. Stir in the honey and salt to taste. Pour into a sterilised jar or glass bottle, seal and keep in the fridge for up to two days.

Immunity tonic

Take this daily as a tablespoonful or a shot. At first it will be a little hard to handle, but persevere and after a week or so, your body will crave the acidity and in turn retain the benefits from all of the incredible herbs and spices.

MAKES 300ML

3 garlic cloves, peeled

1cm knob of fresh ginger, peeled

2.5cm knob of fresh turmeric root, peeled

1 lemon, peeled (keep the peel for another use)

10g fresh horseradish root, peeled

pinch of cayenne pepper

2 tablespoons raw honey

300ml organic raw apple cider vinegar

300ml sterilised glass bottle

Put the garlic, ginger, turmeric, lemon and horseradish through a juice extractor, then mix in all the other ingredients. If you don't have a juicer, grate the garlic and all the roots into a bowl, squeeze in the lemon juice and then mix with all the other ingredients.

Pour into a sterilised glass bottle, seal and label. Store in the fridge and use within 2 weeks. Use as required. Best taken as a small 20ml shot but you can just add a shot to your juice or water.

Immunity tonic is about preventing illness, not curing it. Use food to give your body what it needs to be healthy rather than relying on medicine to fix it.

Dandelion coffee

This is more nutritious than regular coffee, being rich in vitamins A, B, C and D and potassium, iron and zinc. It's also wonderful for those who are sensitive to caffeine but want to feel like they are drinking coffee.

SERVES 2

100g dandelion root
about 500ml boiling water

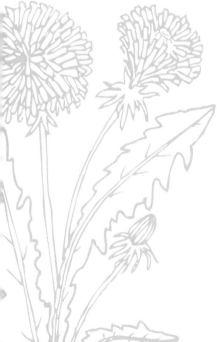

Preheat the oven to 200°C/gas mark 6 and line a baking tray with baking paper.

Wash, dry and cut the dandelion root into pieces. Spread out the pieces on the lined baking tray and bake for 30 minutes. Remove from the oven and leave to cool, then grind to a fine powder in a spice or coffee grinder.

Make the dandelion coffee by putting the ground root into a cafetiere or coffee plunger, then add the boiling water. Leave to infuse for a few minutes, then press down the plunger and pour into mugs. Serve with milk and honey, as desired.

The ground powder can be stored in a jar for up to a month, but it's best made fresh as needed.

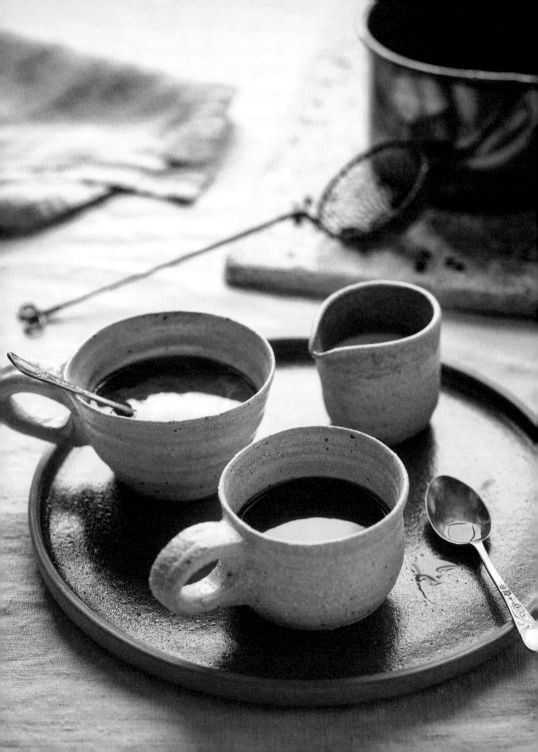

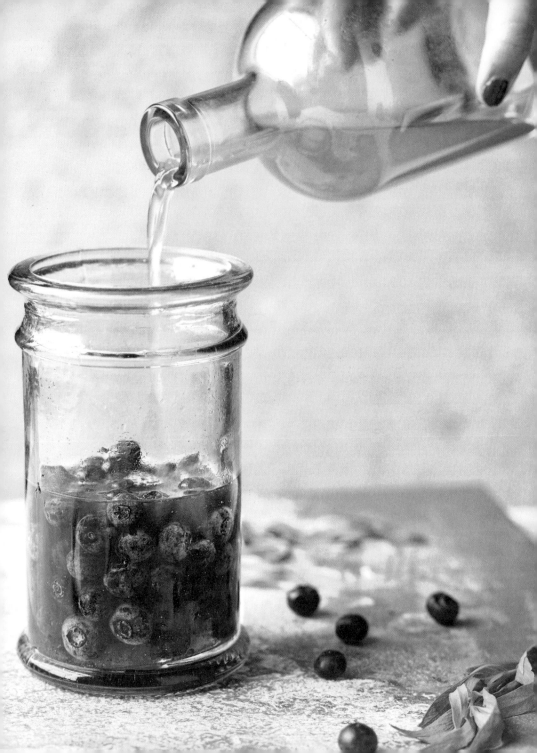

Tarragon & blueberry shrub

Shrub is the name given to a refreshing non-alcoholic drink made by preserving fresh fruit in vinegar, with a little sugar added to offset the tartness. The best part is that you can literally use whatever prepared fresh fruit you have access to, so you can make shrubs whatever the season. The only rule is to ensure the vinegar is above 5 per cent acidity.

MAKES 1 LITRE

750g fresh blueberries
1 litre vinegar (apple cider or
**   kombucha vinegar best)**
large handful of tarragon,
**   leaves picked**
750g granulated sugar

2 sterilised 1 litre jars

Begin by sterilising a 1 litre jar. Add the blueberries to the jar. Heat the vinegar in a saucepan until just before it boils, then pour it over the fruit, leaving at least 2.5cm headspace at the top of the jar. Add the tarragon leaves. Wipe the jar and rim clean, then seal and store in a cool, dark place for 2–4 weeks, shaking occasionally.

After that time, remove the lid and strain the fruit vinegar into a saucepan, discarding the fruit and tarragon. Add the sugar and bring the fruit vinegar to the boil, stirring initially to dissolve the sugar quickly before it boils. Remove from the heat and leave it to cool, then pour into another sterilised jar with a lid. Seal, cool and label.

Store in the fridge for up to 6 months. If any mould develops or fermentation occurs, discard it. Add 1–2 tablespoons of the shrub to a glass of still or sparkling water or to your favourite fruity cocktail.

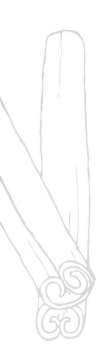

Herbal wine (for health)

Sounds completely contradictory, but with the addition of healing herbs and drunk in moderation, this wine can actually alleviate things such as colds and help with digestion. It's also wonderful to drink heated (like mulled wine), or served over ice in summer.

MAKES 750ML

1 cinnamon stick, crushed
1 tablespoon grated (peeled) fresh ginger
1 teaspoon ground allspice
1 teaspoon dried juniper berries
1 teaspoon cloves
1 teaspoon orange zest
1 teaspoon fresh rosemary leaves
3 bay leaves
1 bottle red wine (shiraz or cabernet sauvignon)
honey, to taste (optional)

sterilised 1 litre jar, plus a sterilised 750ml jar or glass bottle

Put the spices, orange zest and herbs into a 1 litre sterilised jar and pour the red wine over. Seal the jar tightly and shake well. Store in a cool, dry place, out of direct light. Shake every day or so for up to 2 weeks. If you leave the infusions too long, they may be too strong.

After a week, taste and see if you can taste the herbs. If it tastes good, strain out the herbs and spices using a muslin-lined sieve and return to a 750ml sterilised jar or glass bottle. You can add some honey to taste, if you like. Seal, then store in a cool, dark place for up to 6 months. Once opened, use within 2 weeks, and keep in the fridge.

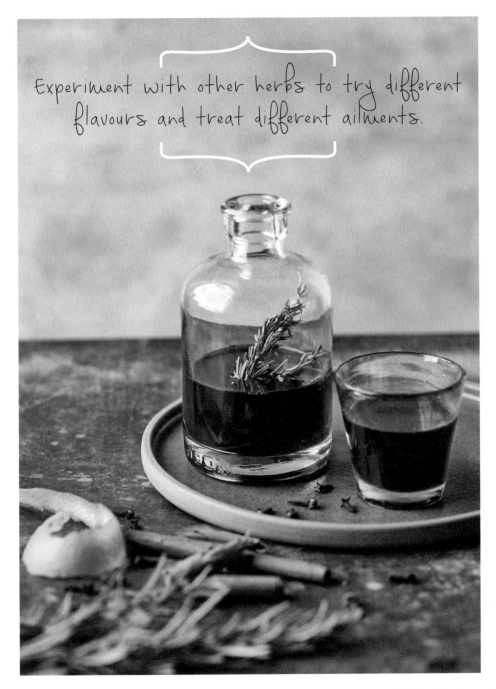

Experiment with other herbs to try different flavours and treat different ailments.

Chapter Three
food

Herby ice lollies

Ice lollies have this incredible power of transporting us to childhood, and for me remind me of super hot summer days running under the garden hose in the backyard with an ice lolly dripping down my arm onto the hot concrete, where it would be quickly eaten by ants. These lollies are less sweet and more about the herbs. Play around with the flavours to suit you. You will need lolly moulds.

FOR 4 YOGURT LOLLIES

450g natural yogurt

2 tablespoons raw honey

plus your choice of one of the
    following:

2 sprigs of lemon balm, leaves
    picked

2 sprigs of basil, leaves picked

2 sprigs of tarragon, leaves picked

2 sprigs of mint, leaves picked

2 sprigs of lavender, flowers picked

FOR 4 SODA WATER LOLLIES

100g raw honey

plus your choice of one or more of
    the following (plus extra for the
    moulds):

4 sprigs of lemon balm, leaves
    picked

4 sprigs of basil, leaves picked

4 sprigs of tarragon, leaves picked

4 sprigs of mint, leaves picked

4 sprigs of lavender, flowers picked

zest and juice of 6 limes

350ml soda water

For the yogurt herb ice lollies, mix the yogurt with the honey in a food-processor. Add your chosen herb leaves or lavender flowers and stir in to combine leaving the leaves whole and flower petals picked, then pour into ice lolly moulds. Push some herbs to the outside of the moulds so that you'll be able to see them. Freeze overnight until firm. These will keep for up to a month in the freezer.

For the soda water ice lollies, pour 200ml tap water into a small saucepan and bring to the boil. Remove from the heat, add the honey and stir until dissolved. Add half of your chosen herb leaves or lavender flowers, return to the heat and simmer for 5 minutes, then remove and leave to infuse for 30 minutes. (This can be prepared the day before and left in the fridge overnight to infuse.)

Pour through a sieve into a jug, squashing the herbs/lavender flowers with the back of a spoon to squeeze out all the juices. Add the lime zest and juice and stir. Add enough soda water to bring the total volume up to 600ml. Add the remaining chosen herb leaves or lavender flowers to the ice lolly moulds, then pour in the liquid. Freeze overnight until firm. These will keep for up to a month in the freezer.

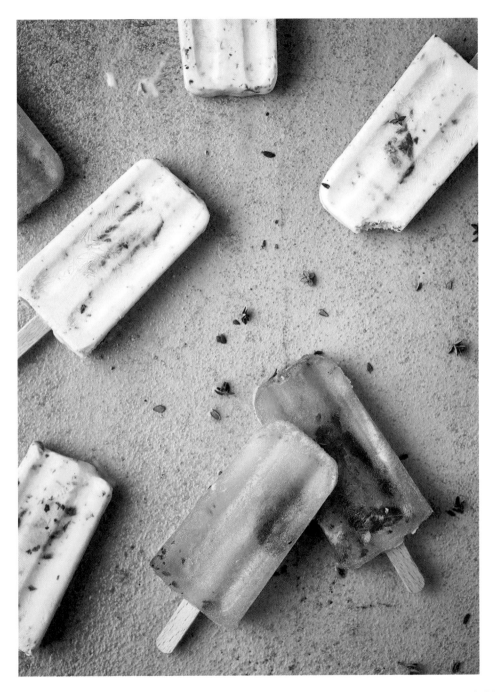

Kefir & lemon verbena bliss balls

I have always wanted to be one of those people that chose a 'bliss ball' over a slice of cake, but had never found one that quite cut the mustard so to speak. Then I tried playing around with a bunch of different recipes and this one was the winner. Goodbye cake, hello bliss balls (most of the time, anyway).

MAKES 8

35g ready-to-eat dried prunes
120g quinoa, cooked and cooled
1 tablespoon macadamia nuts or almond meal
1 tablespoon sunflower seeds
½ tablespoon raw cacao powder
1½ tablespoons maple syrup
30ml milk kefir (optional)
½ teaspoon ground cinnamon
1 tablespoon macadamia nut or almond butter
½ small handful of lemon verbena, fresh and chopped
small handful of freshly picked stinging nettles, finely chopped
1 tablespoon chia seeds
pinch of good-quality salt
pinch of ground cardamom
½ tablespoon coconut oil, melted

to finish
desiccated coconut
Petal Powders (see right)

Blitz the prunes in a food-processor until very finely chopped. Transfer the prunes to a bowl, then add all the remaining ingredients and mix everything together well.

Roll the mixture into walnut-sized balls, then either roll in the desiccated coconut or in the petal powders (I like to roll half the balls in coconut and half in petal powders). Place in an airtight container and store in the fridge. They keep well for up to 2 weeks.

How to make petal powders

You can use petals from any dried edible flowers to make petal powders for natural flavouring and colouring. Calendula, carnations, cornflowers, hibiscus, marigolds, roses and violets all work well — just make sure the petals are crispy dry.

Simply place the dried petals in small batches into a spice grinder and blitz until you get a fine powder. Store in airtight containers.

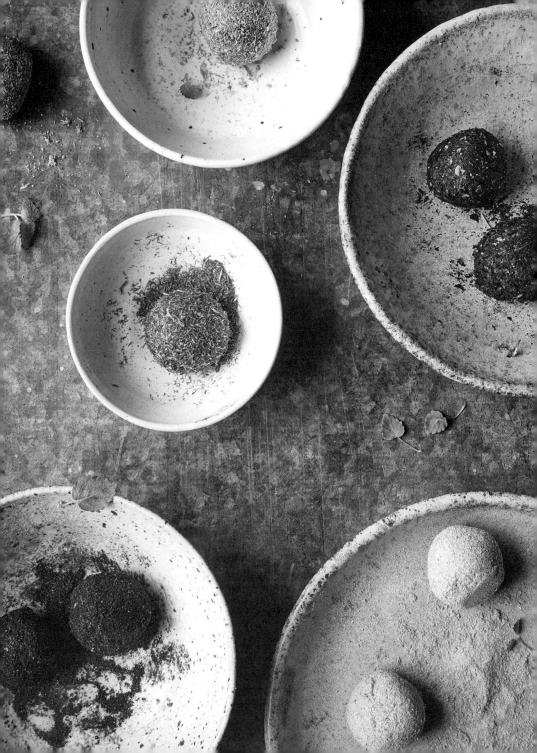

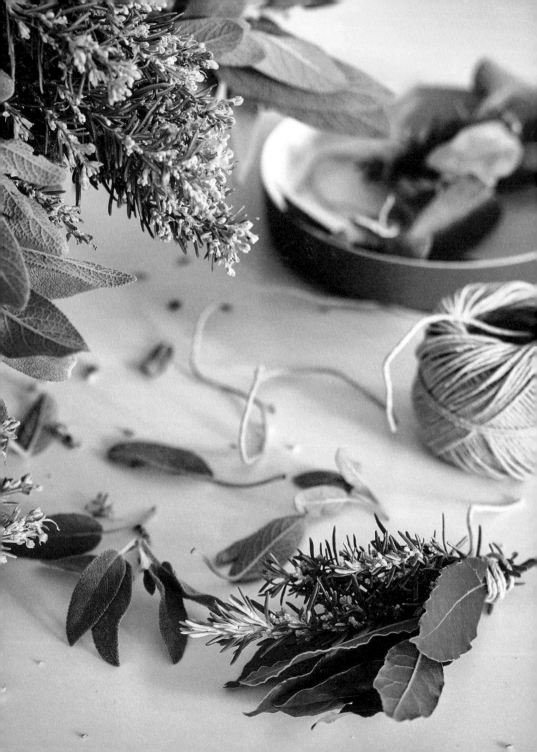

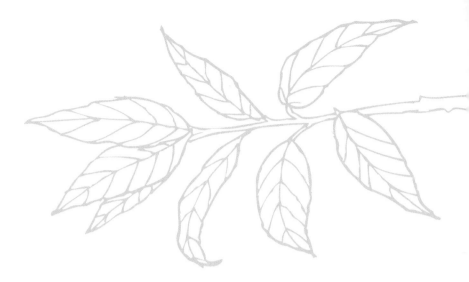

Bouquet garnis

The most traditional bouquet garni comprises parsley, bay leaf and thyme in the ratio eight parts parsley to one part each of bay and thyme. But you should have a garni party and make them any which way you like.

If bouquet garni parties aren't a real thing, they should be!

To make, simply take your chosen herbs, dried or fresh, tie the stalks with a little kitchen string or twine and add to all manner of casseroles, stews, soups and tagines.

Experiment with your preferred combinations – you could try thyme, rosemary and sage; parsley, tarragon and lemon thyme; or mint, basil and parsley.

Herby kraut

Sauerkraut, which in German means sour cabbage, is an age-old method of preserving cabbage and other ingredients by fermentation. 'Kraut' was traditionally prepared to provide vital nutrition in northern Europe during the cold winters when vegetables could not be grown. The same technique is still used today, with more knowledge now of the diverse health benefits associated with fermented foods. For best results, use local, organic or unsprayed ingredients in your kraut. When washing cabbages and other produce for fermenting, I also recommend using filtered water.

MAKES 500G

500g green or red cabbage (keep one intact leaf to act as a bung for the top of the jar)

10g good-quality (not iodised) sea salt (such as Murray River or Maldon sea salt)

100g combined fresh dill and fresh fennel fronds or a pinch of each dried

½ any apple, peeled and grated (optional)

filtered water, if needed

sterilised 500ml jar

Slice the cabbage, cutting against the grain to create thin, medium-length strips, and place in a large bowl. Add your sea salt. With clean hands (but not having used hand sanitiser, as this will kill good bacteria), start to massage the salt into the cabbage for 3–4 minutes. Set aside for the salt to pull the juices from the cabbage. Chop the fresh herbs, ready to be added to the cabbage.

After 5–10 minutes, the salted cabbage will have released more juices and wilted. Continue to massage the cabbage until it has softened and a reasonable amount of brine has been created. Add the herbs and grated apple (if using) to the bowl and mix thoroughly. Now pack into your sterilised jar using your hands to press the cabbage mixture down tightly. You want it packed to within 2–3cm of the top of the jar with brine covering all of it. If the brine doesn't quite cover it, top up with a little filtered water.

Fold a small portion of the reserved cabbage leaf and place on top of the cabbage mixture to keep it submerged in the brine, but ensure there is still room to put a lid on. Wipe any bits from the rim of the jar using kitchen paper and put on the lid. Leave to ferment at room temperature for at least 4 days and up to 3 weeks. For a ferment using this technique, I find 7–10 days works well.

Remember that gas (carbon dioxide) is released during the fermentation process, so it is important to open the lid to 'burp' the jar every day or two to release the gases, but be quick to reseal it so oxygen doesn't get a chance to sneak in and spoil your ferment. So you will literally open the lid but not take it off or lift it up. I suggest 'burping' on days 3, 5 and 7. After this, remove the cabbage leaf and taste the kraut. If you are happy with it, replace the lid, refrigerate and enjoy within 2 months.

Herby pesto

The most fabulous way of all time to use up leftover herbs is to make a pesto. You could also use carrot tops – I hate to throw anything away, so if I buy a bunch of carrots I'll use up the tops in a pesto.

SERVES 4

3 tablespoons pine nuts or almonds
50g basil, roughly chopped
large handful each of tarragon and mint
2 garlic cloves, minced
zest and juice of 1 lemon
3 tablespoons grated Parmesan cheese
olive oil
salt and freshly ground black pepper, to taste

Toast the nuts in a dry frying pan over a medium heat until they turn golden. Watch carefully and move them around the pan while they are cooking as they can burn easily. Tip onto a plate and leave to cool.

Add the herbs and pine nuts to a food-processor and blitz until smooth. Add the garlic and lemon zest and juice and blitz again for a few seconds. Now add the Parmesan and then, with the processor running, add enough olive oil until you have the consistency you like for your pesto. Season to taste with salt and pepper and blitz again for a few more seconds.

Spoon into an airtight container or jar and store in the fridge for up to a week (or freeze in ice cube trays for up to 3 months). Add more oil if it becomes too dry.

Wild green salsa

I like to nickname this the all-purpose green sauce. It honestly
works in everything, from pasta (as a pesto) to toasted cheese
sandwiches, on meat and stirred through roast veggies. Jam-
packed with good things for your body and great things for
your taste buds, too.

MAKES 1 SERVING

1 garlic clove, peeled
1 tablespoon capers, rinsed
    and drained
2 canned anchovy fillets, drained
2 handfuls of flat-leaf parsley
handful of rocket leaves
small handful of lemon balm leaves
small handful of wild garlic leaves
    or flowers
small handful of freshly picked
    stinging nettles
1 tablespoon apple cider vinegar
    or lemon juice
about 6 tablespoons olive oil
salt and freshly ground black pepper

Place the garlic, capers, anchovies,
parsley, rocket, lemon balm, wild
garlic and nettles in a food-
processor and blitz until finely
chopped (or you can crush the
garlic and finely chop the other
ingredients by hand).

Transfer the mixture to a bowl and
stir in the vinegar. Drizzle in enough
olive oil, stirring continuously, until
you have a fairly thick consistency.
Season well with salt and pepper.
Use immediately or store in an airtight
jar in the fridge for up to 5 days.

Drying herbs

Drying out fresh herbs is an amazing way to make the most of seasonal gluts and can add a huge amount of flavour to many a dish. Let's not forget they have been used for centuries in tinctures and tonics, and for general health and wellbeing.

Pick your herbs into individual leaves. Put some sheets of kitchen paper on trays and lay out the individual leaves separately, spreading them apart so the air can circulate. The paper helps to draw any moisture away from the leaves.

Find a place out of draughts to dry the leaves, preferably inside. Near a window is good to give them sufficient sunlight for drying – direct sunlight dries them faster, but they fade a little.

Leave them for 1–2 days. Check on them as they may dry sooner, depending on your home: they like dry heat, no humidity. You will know when they are dry as they feel like tissue paper and wrinkle up a little.

Once the leaves have dried, play around with mixtures to make the perfect Italian-style herb addition to your meals. I love using rosemary, thyme and oregano together in equal parts. Store them in small jars or airtight containers, crumbling or gently crushing them as you go – they will last for ages and the flavour is stronger than when using fresh herbs.

Drying in bunches

Bunches of drying woody herbs (such as rosemary, thyme, lavender or sage) look pretty tied to a shelf or hanging above your oven. Simply gather your fresh herbs, tie a bunch together and hang upside down out of direct sunlight. If you want to speed up the process, you may be able to dry them outside in warm (not humid) air and bring them inside when dried. If you live in a humid country though, dry them inside in a dry place. Leave them hanging and snip off the leaves as and when needed.

Dried herbs look gorgeous
hanging in your kitchen and also help
to keep little bugs away.

Herb-infused oils

Herb-infused oils are not just great for cooking, they also make lovely gifts and can be used as massage oil or added to the bath (although avoid the garlic and chilli in these cases!). You can use any oil you like for this, though it's best to use one you like to cook with.

Before you start, you need to dry out your chosen fresh herbs for at least 12 hours to stop them going rancid.

Sterilise and thoroughly dry a large jar or glass bottle. Fill it with the herbs, either on their own or along with whole dried or fresh chillies, whole (peeled) garlic or some edible flowers, depending on what you want to use the oil for.

Slowly pour oil over the herbs and spices/flowers. Use a skewer or similar to move the herbs around to ensure no air pockets remain.

Add enough oil to completely cover all the herbs, filling your vessel right up to the brim.

Tightly seal the jar or bottle. Place it on a sunny windowsill to 2 weeks, shaking every couple of days. This is called solar infusion.

After that time, strain the oil into sterilised glass bottles through a muslin-lined sieve. Give the herbs a squish in the sieve before discarding. Seal and label your bottles. Store in a cool, dark place for up to 2 years. Once opened, use within 6 months.

Adding a few drops of Vitamin E oil to your herb oil will help to prolong its shelf life.

Freezing herbs in oil

Pick off individual fresh herb leaves and place a few into ice cube trays. Cover with the oil of your choice, using a ratio of one part herbs to three parts oil. Freeze until solid, then simply pop out a couple of cubes when cooking. You can use these cubes straight from frozen, simply popped out into a medium-hot frying pan.

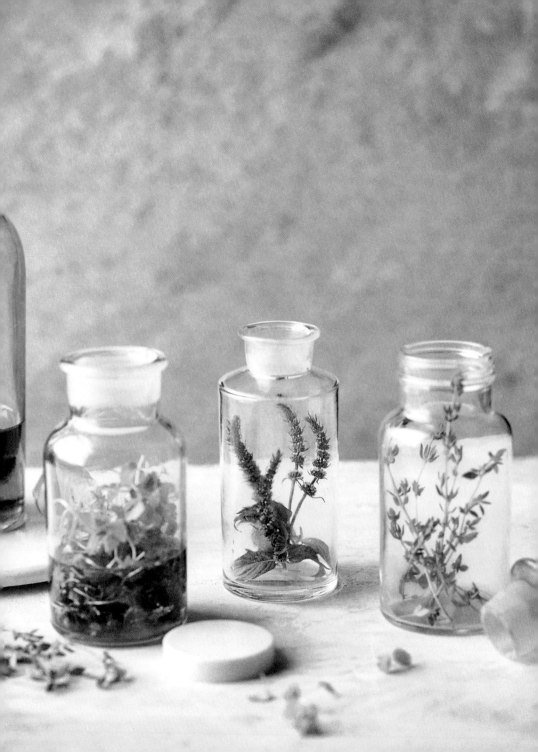

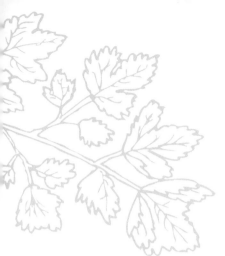

Herb butter

My favourite kind of butter is the one I churn myself, and the easiest way to do it in 5 minutes or less (depending on your muscle power) is using a jar and a marble. It's great fun for kids (and big kids too). When you have an excess glut of herbs, it's the perfect time to make butter.

MAKES 250G

250ml organic single cream, at
    room temperature
pinch of salt, plus extra to taste
a handful of fresh herbs (such as
    parsley, coriander, mint, sage,
    rosemary, thyme or lemon
    balm, or a combination of
    sage and lavender or rosemary,
    parsley, sage and thyme), finely
    chopped

1 litre jar (choose a strong jar with
    thick glass or, failing that, an
    old plastic milk bottle – just
    avoid anything with thin glass
    as the marble could crack it)
1 large glass marble
bowl of cold water with ice cubes in

Put the cream and the pinch of salt into the jar and add the marble. Shake with the marble for about 3 minutes, or until the cream first looks softly whipped, then becomes stiff. You will hear the marble at first, then as the cream stiffens you won't hear it. What will happen from here is as you keep shaking, all of a sudden you will hear the marble again as the buttermilk begins to separate from the cream. Keep shaking until the buttermilk separates. Once it does, strain off the buttermilk (use it for something else). Give the jar another shake or two, take the butter out and squeeze out any more buttermilk.

Put the butter into the bowl of iced water and use your hands to massage the remaining buttermilk out – you need to remove it all, otherwise it will sour the butter. Wash the butter a couple of times, dipping it in and out of the water, then pat it dry and place in a bowl.

Sprinkle over some salt, mix in your chopped herbs and mould into whatever shape you like. Put into an airtight container or wrap in clingfilm and keep in the fridge for up to 5 days.

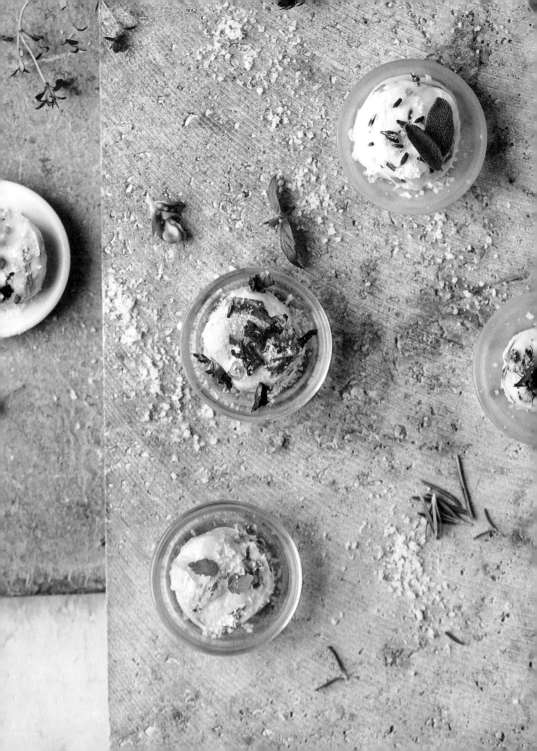

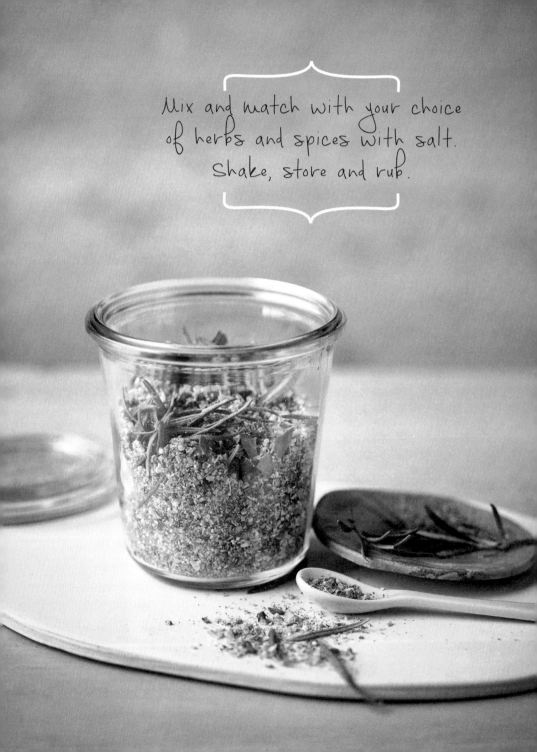

Mix and match with your choice of herbs and spices with salt. Shake, store and rub.

Herby salt rub

Turn boring meat and veg into a restaurant quality meal simply by adding some herbs and spices. Make a jar of this to keep in your pantry and use it on everything. This is another great little jar that makes a lovely gift.

MAKES 1 SMALL JAR

1½ tablespoons fresh rosemary
   leaves
1 tablespoon dried chilli flakes
1 tablespoon garlic powder
1 tablespoons whole yellow
   mustard seeds, crushed
2 tablespoons paprika
2 tablespoons fresh thyme leaves
1 tablespoon dried oregano
2 dried bay leaves, crushed
125g good-quality sea salt

sterilised small jar with lid or
   airtight container

Place all the ingredients in the jar. Put on the lid and shake until the ingredients are combined, then store in a cool, dry place for up to a year.

Use as a rub or a sprinkle on raw meats and veggies before roasting, as required.

Resources

Below are just some of the fantastic suppliers you can source your ingredients and equipment from.

HERBS – WORLDWIDE
Flora Export S.G. Israel
www.flora-sg.com

HERBS – UK & IRELAND
Riverford
www.riverford.co.uk
Abel & Cole
www.abelandcole.co.uk
Greens of Devon
www.greensofdevon.com
Herbs Unlimited
www.herbsunlimited.co.uk
Organic Herb Trading
www.organicherbtrading.com

HERBS – AUSTRALIA
Australian Fresh Leaf Herbs
www.freshleaf.com.au
Sprout House Farms
www.sprouthousefarms.com.au
Flowerdale Farm
www.flowerdalefarm.com.au
All Rare Herbs
www.allrareherbs.com.au

DRIED HERBS, SPICES & FLOWERS –
WORLDWIDE
Herb Affair
www.herbaffair.com

DRIED HERBS, SPICES & FLOWERS – UK
& IRELAND
Pestle Herbs
www.pestleherbs.co.uk

DRIED HERBS, SPICES & FLOWERS –
AUSTRALIA
Austral Herbs
www.australherbs.com.au

BOTTLES AND JARS, PACKAGING AND
DRIED INGREDIENTS – WORLDWIDE
New Directions Australia
www.newdirections.com.au
Amazon
www.amazon.com

Index

Acknowledgements

Firstly to my family. My mum and dad have always supported me and I love that they sit in what my dad calls his 'proud chair' because of the path I am on. All I have ever wanted was to make them and my brothers proud. So to you my small family and the rest of my big extended family, especially its oh so wonderful leader my nan (and great grandmother Lil). To all of you, Sarah, Nigel, Paul, Mark, Kylie, Skye, Angie, Bec, Harry, Nicole, Yasmin, Sam, Teryn, Ashleigh, Caitlyn, Liam, Brad and Taylah and then the rest of our little family Emma, Koen and my godsons Charlie and Rory. You are all everything to me. As are you Damien, my love. Thank you for putting up with our home looking like a constant laboratory and test kitchen. To my friends who have supported me for decades.

To Kyle. I have no words to express how grateful I am to you. To our new Octopus family, here is to a long journey making beautiful and meaningful books together. To my team. The A team. Tara, the most incredible Editor a girl could ask for. Your patience, generosity and passion for these next books made them what they are. Nassima. Thank you for making my recipes and creations come to life. I only hope we work on many a more things together. Rachel. No words can thank you enough for being the most incredible partner in crime styling these books and seeing inside my messy brain. You are so immensely talented and I am so grateful. Agathe, Laura and the rest of the team. High fives all round! To all of the people in my work world who have taught me so very much over the years. Thank you. There is no way I would be where I am without you teaching me everything I know. Last but not at all least, to all of you who bought this book. Massive gratitude from the bottom of my heart.